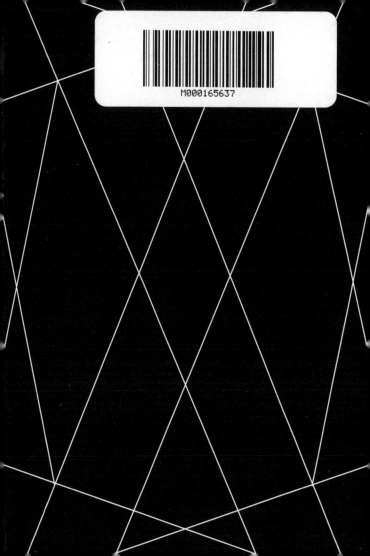

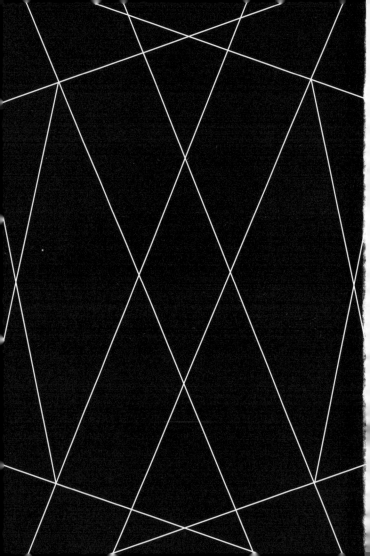

YOU'RE NOT ALONE

Good Advice and Kind Words for When You Feel Lonely

DEBBI MARCO

YOU'RE NOT ALONE

An Hachette UK Company
www.hachette.co.uk

Vie Books, an imprint of Summersdale Publishers Ltd
Part of Octopus Publishing Group Limited
Carmelite House
50 Victoria Embankment
LONDON
EC4Y 0DZ
UK

www.summersdale.com

Printed and bound in China

ISBN: 978-1-80007-394-4

Substantial discounts on bulk quantities of Summersdale books are available to corporations, professional associations and other organizations. For details contact general enquiries: telephone: +44 (0) 1243 771107 or email: enquiries@summersdale.com.

Disclaimer
This book is not intended as a substitute for the medical advice of a doctor or physician. If you are experiencing problems with your health, it is always best to follow the advice of a medical professional.

Contents

INTRODUCTION

Loneliness feels different to everyone who is experiencing it. You could feel lonely because you haven't seen or spoken to anyone in days, or it could be that you're surrounded by people at home and at work but still feel lonely. Feeling misunderstood or not being listened to can exacerbate disconnection. The UK Office of National Statistics says loneliness is on the increase, and it can have a huge impact on our mental well-being. However, it's important to recognize there is a big difference between being alone and feeling lonely. For this reason, learning how to enjoy your own company and spend time on your own is vital.

This book will help you identify the reasons you might be feeling lonely and what you can do about it. By examining the smaller elements of your life, such as your diet or your work/life balance, and learning how to create meaningful connections with others, you can learn when you want to be alone and when you prefer to be with others. You will also uncover skills to help you avoid feeling lonely as well as how to be happy and at ease with the most important person in your life – yourself.

BEING ALONE HAS
NOTHING TO DO WITH
HOW MANY PEOPLE
ARE AROUND.

RICHARD YATES

WHY AM I LONELY?

There are many reasons why you might develop feelings of loneliness and everyone's experience is unique. It may be that you aren't interacting with as many people during the day or it isn't currently possible to fulfil your desire for an intimate social connection. Whatever the reason, know that many people feel lonely and it's completely natural to do so. This chapter will help you identify the reasons why you may be feeling this way and share small but significant techniques that can help to change this.

ARE YOU ALONE OR LONELY?

It might seem like an obvious distinction but being alone is very different to feeling lonely. Many people enjoy spending time alone. It gives them the opportunity to switch off, recharge and do something they like without having to make compromises with other people. Ultimately, there are a lot of positives to having time on your own, and, throughout this book, you'll learn how to optimize this alone time. Feelings of loneliness, however, are very different and shouldn't be confused with having time to yourself. Loneliness is subjective and can result from a lack of close social contact or affection. Bear in mind, people seek different levels of human connections, and this can vary for each person. If you're feeling lonely, the first thing you need to do is identify what is missing or out of balance in your life. Only then can you figure out how to fill your life to make it richer.

FEELING LONELY IS
FINE. STAYING THIS WAY
FOREVER IS NOT.

MAXIME LAGACÉ

Being alone allows you the space you need to discover yourself

YOU'RE NOT ALONE

While it's easy to feel you're the only one battling feelings of loneliness, the truth is you have more company than you think. A loneliness epidemic has been building for years, and the Covid-19 pandemic has only made these feelings more prevalent. An increased number of people working from home has reduced the connections that come with an office-based work life. And while social media appears to offer connectivity, it is just as easy to feel as though you're not part of the conversation. By acknowledging that it's normal to feel lonely sometimes, you may feel more confident in tackling those feelings.

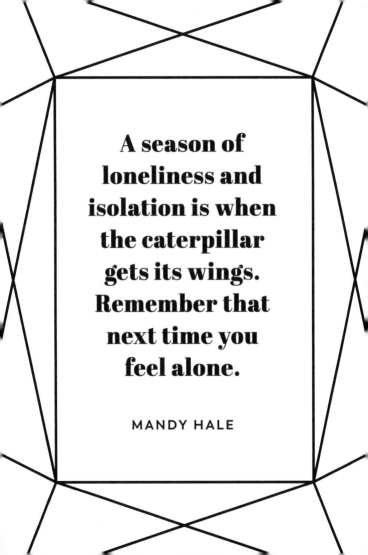

A season of
loneliness and
isolation is when
the caterpillar
gets its wings.
Remember that
next time you
feel alone.

MANDY HALE

Get to the root of the problem

Give yourself some time to figure out why you're feeling lonely. Could it be that you're not happy in your job, your relationship isn't quite right, or you don't feel supported by loved ones? Perhaps your loneliness is the result of a recent house move or having split up with a partner? Maybe your best friend has moved away, or a close relative has died. Sometimes the reason behind loneliness isn't so obvious. In those instances, talking to friends or family about how you feel may help to identify the causes. Alternatively, you could write down your feelings in a notebook and pay attention to recurrent themes. You might find it's due to more than one thing. Some issues may even be interlinked. If this is the case, take it a step at a time by picking one thing that you feel more confident in tackling. For example, if you've moved to a new area, you could join a walking group which would help you get to know your new home and open you up to making friends.

Sometimes it's nice to be alone

Plan ahead

Feelings of loneliness can sometimes be exacerbated by the time of year. For example, some people find Christmas lonely as this is when people traditionally spend time with family and friends. It doesn't help that the weather is often cold and dreary too. Try to pre-empt seasonal loneliness by scheduling an activity you enjoy – such as preparing your favourite meal or taking a long hike. It could mean treating yourself to a trip to the cinema or theatre. If you do have someone you can spend the holidays with, reach out in advance to see whether they want to get together.

IT'S HEALTHY
TO SPEND
TIME ALONE

Find your tribe

Are you a single parent? Maybe you're struggling with your mental health. Or perhaps you have a mobility issue that might stop you from socializing as easily. A simple online search can direct you to local organizations or community groups who bring like-minded people together. If you feel comfortable, offer to meet with group leaders or join a group get-together. While you might feel alone right now, you can be sure there are others out there who feel the way you do. This is a great opportunity to find them.

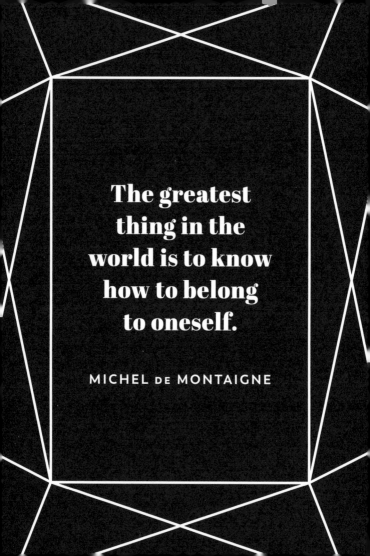

The greatest
thing in the
world is to know
how to belong
to oneself.

MICHEL DE MONTAIGNE

TAKE YOUR TIME

While you may have made the decision to tackle your loneliness, it is unlikely that your social interactions will change overnight. The chances are that a forced busy schedule wouldn't be very enjoyable – especially if it doesn't come naturally to you. Instead, tune into your feelings and don't push yourself too fast. Perhaps encourage yourself to meet new people or reignite an old connection once a week or once a fortnight. Relationships, at least the ones worth having, can take months or years to build. Give any new connections time to grow slowly and organically.

BOOST YOUR CONFIDENCE

It might seem like a separate issue, but often those who struggle with loneliness lack the confidence to reach out and connect with others. This could be for many reasons, including that you may struggle to believe you are worth connecting with. Start boosting your self-worth by writing a love letter to yourself. Reminisce about times when you've helped others, achieved something you're proud of, or done something you've been scared of. You could even pop a stamp on the letter and post it to yourself – after all, it's nice to receive mail that isn't a bill.

Another trick is to keep a journal of all the times you've done something worthy. It could be anything from giving up your seat on the bus, donating to charity or making someone laugh. Try to write in it every day. You'll soon see what an amazing person you are and that you are worth spending time with. With this new-found confidence, you might even attract the connections and relationships that you're seeking.

IT'S OKAY TO
BE MADLY
IN LOVE
WITH YOURSELF

IF YOU MAKE
FRIENDS WITH
YOURSELF, YOU
WILL NEVER
BE ALONE.

MAXWELL MALTZ

LEARN FROM THE PAST

Ask yourself why you are feeling lonely right now. Has something changed recently? Can you trace your life back to a time when you didn't feel lonely? What was happening then? Consider whether there is anything you can learn from your younger self and the time when you felt less lonely. If you've always felt lonely, that's okay. There are still lessons you can learn. What have you always done that is the same? Is it time to try something new such as changing your job or joining a club?

Embrace the beauty of a journey taken alone

IT'S OKAY TO ASK FOR HELP

An overwhelming feeling of loneliness is often a sign that something else isn't quite right. It could be that you are suffering with grief from a bereavement or the break-up of a relationship. Perhaps the strain from a job or your everyday responsibilities is taking its toll. Maybe you have money worries that mean you're not free to take positive actions. No matter what the deeper issue is, there's no need to feel ashamed that you're not coping on your own. There are plenty of charities and healthcare professionals who can help you find a happier new you. Search the internet to see if there is a local charity that can help with your specific problem. If not, make an appointment with your doctor. Be truthful about how you're feeling, and they should be able to direct you to someone who can help. Asking for help and taking that first step towards a happier, more positive life shows strength. Check out the final chapter of this book for more tips and advice on how to find the help you need.

Learn
to love
your own
company

BE KIND TO YOUR BODY

Have you noticed it is pretty hard to feel sad when you're dancing round your kitchen to your favourite tune? That's because endorphins, the feel-good hormones, are flooding your body. And there are plenty of other ways of looking after your body that can lift your mood and help ease overwhelming feelings of loneliness and despair. While being fit and healthy won't fix all your problems; it will definitely put you on track to start tackling them the right way.

Move in
the morning

Whether you prefer a yogic sun salutation or a bracing jog, starting your day with some form of movement is great for getting your heart pumping and oxygen flowing through your body. By shaking off a potentially sluggish start, you'll be primed to face any problems that may come your way. And while you may not always feel like jumping out of bed to start exercising, you can help yourself by laying out your kit the night before – a gentle nudge that can make it easier to crawl out from under your snuggly duvet. So, whether you choose a bracing cold water swim, a brisk walk, a gentle stretching session or something else, endeavour to keep moving and see how good it makes you feel afterwards. Once you start noticing the improvement in your body, you might even look forward to getting up and out each day. And if you can make this morning movement a habit, there's no doubt you'll be reaping the rewards in no time.

Slow and steady

If you think that exercise means sweating it out at the gym or sprinting round a running track, think again. Slow exercise can be just as beneficial for the body. Not only does it reduce the risk of injury, it can also help strengthen your mind. The flow of yoga, the precise moves of Pilates or the gentle repetition of swimming laps, for example, can often be just the thing you need to get your thoughts in order, without breaking a sweat.

I WILL SHOW
MYSELF LOVE,
KINDNESS AND
ACCEPTANCE

GET GROUNDED

Step outside, slip off your shoes and peel off your socks. Now sink your feet into some lush green grass, a shallow river or some grainy sand – whatever is nearby. Focus on the sensation of the ground beneath your feet. Feel your toes grasp whatever surface you're standing on, even if it's just a pavement. Focus on the sensation against your skin. Is it cool, hot, dry or wet? Is the ground firm or is it squishing through your toes? You can even shut your eyes if you feel safe – be careful not to lose your balance – and breathe deeply, enjoying that sense of being truly grounded.

Feeling physically connected to the earth can help mentally connect you and stop your mind wandering off into unhelpful and negative thought patterns. When you're ready to go on with your day, try to carry this feeling of being grounded with you and return to it whenever you're feeling a bit wobbly.

Clear
your clutter

It may seem like a small issue, but when your living space is cluttered with heaps of laundry, piles of books and dirty plates, it can really affect how you feel day-to-day. So, why not make a date to have a clear-out and tidy up. Start small – even if it's just sorting through one pile of laundry or one drawer. Be strong in your method by throwing out anything broken, giving away things you don't want and keeping only what you love. As you create a neater space, you might find yourself more in control of your mind too.

ALONE TIME IS WHEN I DISTANCE MYSELF FROM THE VOICES OF THE WORLD, SO I CAN HEAR MY OWN.

OPRAH WINFREY

AXE THE ALCOHOL

Alcohol has long been a social crutch when we're feeling less than confident in social situations and it can also be used to boost us after a stressful day, with many uncorking a bottle of wine to wind down after work. However, while alcohol can seem to help you forget less welcome feelings; it is also a known depressant – meaning it's likely you will feel worse the next day. Rather than turning to alcohol, challenge yourself to drink less. It might seem scary at first, but when you realize you can get through a tough day without an alcohol-filled glass in your hand, you'll know you're capable of pretty much anything.

Be stronger than your strongest excuse

SORT OUT YOUR SLEEP

Good quality sleep is one of the most important gifts you can give yourself as it will help boost your mental and physical health. Of course, if you're suffering from insomnia, you might need to seek professional help, but there are always things you can do to help improve your evening rest. Start by switching off all screens at least an hour before you intend to go to bed as the blue light they create is known to interfere with your body's ability to produce the sleep hormone melatonin. Before you head to bed, try taking a warm bath with calming essential oils. Then instead of scrolling through Twitter, read a book or listen to a meditation podcast. If possible, keep all your tech charging in a different room and invest in an old-fashioned alarm clock so you don't need your phone. If you're really struggling to feel comfortable, try a weighted blanket. You can use it to relax before bed or even sleep with it as the pressure is similar to a hug – and who doesn't want one of those as you drift off to sleep?

FEED FUTURE YOU

There will always be days when you can't be bothered to cook, and that greasy takeaway is looking like a good choice. Only, you already know you'll end up feeling bloated and unhealthy if that's what you choose. But what if you had a fairy "food mother" who had stocked your freezer with some healthy options? Great news – you do, and it is you! Next time you're cooking up your favourite dish, be it a chilli, curry or lasagne, double up your quantities and pop half in the freezer for another day. You'll thank yourself later.

NEVER BE AFRAID
TO SIT AWHILE
AND THINK.

LORRAINE HANSBERRY

Forest bathing

Spending time in natural surroundings – such as a lush green forest – is an activity known as "forest bathing" and is proven to boost your mental health. It might sound slightly strange at first but letting the natural beauty of the branches and tree canopies wash over you while you take in the intricate details of your surroundings is an incredibly relaxing and life-affirming process. Take time to notice the patterns of dappled daylight, tune into bird calls and breathe in the fresh air. This simple activity can leave you feeling intrinsically connected to the earth – and far from alone.

WHEN YOU ARE ALONE, TAKE THE TIME TO STRENGTHEN YOUR MIND

Walk on the mindful side

How often have you gone for a walk and not had your phone in your hand? Perhaps now is the time to try a mindful walk where you have nothing to distract you from the sights, smells and sounds that are all around. It doesn't matter if you're in a city or the country; there's still plenty to appreciate as long as you're paying attention. By leaving your phone behind, you'll be able to focus on your surroundings, and being in the present moment.

Begin your journey by letting someone know where you plan to go and when you will return. Then, as you set off, be sure to absorb all the different colours around you, listening for the sounds of nature or the buzz of busy roads in the distance. Is there anything you now notice that you've never spotted before? By immersing yourself completely in your surroundings, you'll find you are able to switch off from your worries. And hopefully, when you log back into your life, you'll feel like you've been rebooted to focus on things with a fresh energy.

LOVE ON
A PLATE

Food can play such an important part in how we feel about ourselves. Sometimes, it feels as though eating a comforting meal every night is self-love, but eating fresh, healthy and nutritious food is more likely to help you feel better – both physically and mentally. One easy way to do this is to "eat the rainbow". This means you eat a range of fresh fruit and vegetables of different colours over the day, absorbing the healthy vitamins and minerals that come with them. By taking the time to seek out these foods, you can ensure you're getting all the nutrients you need.

Of course, you can eat less healthy foods too, but as an occasional treat rather than an everyday occurrence. After a few weeks you should notice you feel less sluggish, your skin is clearer, and you have the energy to take on any obstacles that life throws at you.

For a tasty and energy-boosting smoothie, try throwing some oats, a banana and some frozen berries, along with a handful of spinach and some milk (or a milk substitute), into a blender.

WHAT A LOVELY
SURPRISE TO FINALLY
DISCOVER HOW
UNLONELY BEING
ALONE CAN BE.

ELLEN BURSTYN

Allow yourself time alone in order to gather strength

Cut the caffeine

While a daily cup of coffee has proven health benefits, too much caffeine can make you feel jittery, irritable and create a low mood, which is not what you need when you're trying to combat feelings of loneliness. If you find yourself drinking copious amounts of tea and coffee throughout the day, it might be time to make a change. Try switching to herbal teas or even just plain water after midday. Add a slice of lemon or a few mint leaves to pep up your drink – you should soon notice your mood swings lessen, and your sleep improves.

Never be
afraid
to spend
time in
your own
company

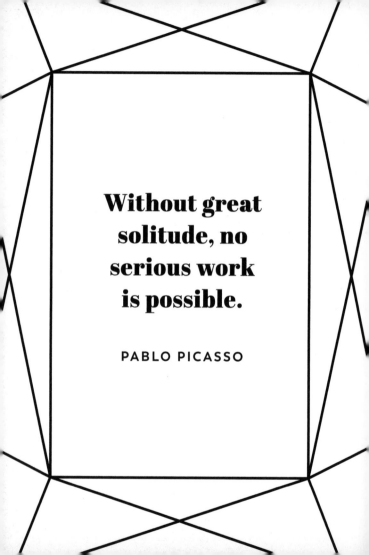

Without great solitude, no serious work is possible.

PABLO PICASSO

LIFE BEGINS
AT THE END
OF YOUR
COMFORT ZONE

SWITCH UP YOUR SNACKS

Grabbing a chocolate bar or can of soda from a vending machine might give you a quick and temporary pick-me-up but you'll soon find yourself in a post-sugar-high slump. This rollercoaster of energy highs and lows can impact your mental health as well as your energy levels. Instead, try to even out your sugar levels with some clever snacking by grabbing a handful of nuts, eating a banana or spreading peanut butter on slices of apple. These will provide slow-release energy and keep you on a more even keel.

BE KIND TO
YOUR MIND

Often you can be your own worst critic, saying things to yourself you'd never say to a friend or loved one. Now is the time to stop berating yourself for bad habits, jobs not done or self-perceived failings. This chapter will provide you with lots of self-care tips and tricks to help you become your own best friend. By learning how to nurture your mind and love yourself, you'll hopefully find the confidence to tackle your feelings of loneliness.

AND BREATHE...

You may think breathing is something you don't need to practise, but actually when you're stressed or feeling nervous, your breathing is the first thing to change. It can get very shallow and cause a tightness in your chest, which leaves you feeling panicky and unable to react calmly. Spending just a few minutes each day learning how to slow down your breath and ensuring you breathe deeply will help you keep calm when it matters most.

Try "square breathing". Imagine you are tracing your finger up one side of a square. As you do so breathe in for the count of four. Now trace your finger along the top of the square as you hold your breath for four. Move your finger down the other side of the square and breathe out for four. Trace the final side of the square and hold your breath for the count of four again. Repeat the exercise until you feel calmer. Now, if you're feeling stressed or your breathing gets shallow, use this simple exercise to regain control and calm your mind.

MAKE TIME TO MEDITATE

Meditation is an ancient practice that will see you focus your attention onto a single thing for an extended period, such as your breath, the wind in the trees or the feel of warm water on your hands. It can be a powerful tool to help draw your awareness away from your thoughts and stop you ruminating on negative feelings of loneliness or letting a low mood spiral out of control. Meditation can be practised at any time. Use an app to help you get the hang of it.

PRACTISE
BEING KIND
TO YOURSELF

Amazing aromatherapy

Ever noticed how a certain smell can remind you of a childhood memory or a person you know? This is because smell directly affects the part of your brain that regulates emotions. As well as triggering memories, aromatherapy can help to reduce stress. Experiment to find out which aromatherapy oil is right for you. Lavender is great for relaxation and sandalwood helps to ease anxiety. Jasmine can aid depression, and orange will help focus a wandering mind. Add a few drops to a fragrance-free base oil or to a warm bath. Then breathe deeply and allow your senses to be enveloped and soothed.

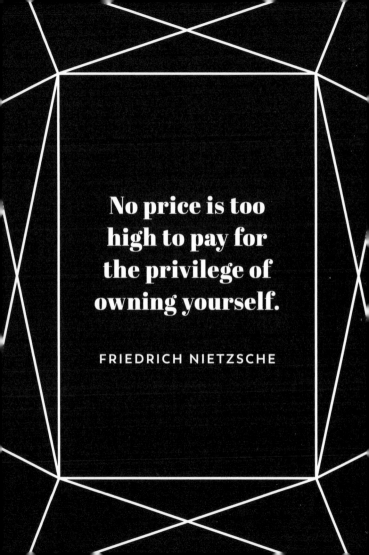

No price is too high to pay for the privilege of owning yourself.

FRIEDRICH NIETZSCHE

Collect your compliments

Any time someone gives you a compliment – whether it's for your beautifully baked bread, a work presentation well done or a particularly well-thought-out outfit – make a note of it. Literally. Either write it down in a specially chosen notebook or on a scrap of paper that you can pop in a jar. Now, whenever you're feeling down on yourself, lacking in connection or unnoticed by others, either at work or in your personal life, you can go back and reread all those small wins. Take the time to examine those words carefully, noting the fondness and goodwill that has gone into each uplifting word. By reading the positive language others use to describe you, you'll experience a boost to your mood and feel reconnected with the person who gave the compliment. This is evidence that you are admired, cared for and even loved. Allow yourself to be comforted by each and every compliment, and, in turn, hopefully, you will feel less alone.

Manifest your confidence

It may seem as though everyone else is confident and happy all the time, but logically, this just can't be true. They're simply better at carrying on when they're not feeling their best. You, too, can achieve this by adopting a more positive or confident persona. Soon, you'll start to find elements of your persona will come true. The lines between what you're pretending to be and how you feel will blur to manifest a genuine mental strength. Watch as your new-found confidence starts attracting more people into your life.

It's okay to choose peace over company

RELY ON RESILIENCE

It's not easy to keep on moving forward when you're feeling low or lonely, but if you can manage to keep putting one foot in front of the other, it can really help lift your spirits.

Keeping going when life feels tough is what resilience is about, and by gradually building up your personal resilience you'll find you are better able to cope with the challenges that life throws at you. Plus, once you realize that you can do difficult things, your self-esteem will grow and you'll find yourself moving towards a more positive outlook. But don't aim too high. The secret with resilience is to build it up like a muscle. Start small. Perhaps set the goal of attending a social event you were reluctant to go to, or maybe look for a new club or evening class to join. It will feel tough at first, but once you've achieved these smaller wins, you'll start to believe in yourself more and more. Soon you'll feel empowered and ready to make the changes in your life that you really want to see.

It's okay
to take
a break

SEEK THOSE WHO FAN YOUR FLAMES.

RUMI

DETOX YOUR RELATIONSHIPS

When it comes to relationships, quality is always more important than quantity. Sometimes when you're worried about not having enough people in your life, it can feel necessary to hang onto the wrong ones. If you have people around you who make you feel less than great, you should consider getting rid of them ASAP. Remember, your friends and partners should always be the cheerleaders in your life even though you may occasionally disagree or argue. Once you've culled any toxic friendships, you'll have more time and energy to find the friends who are right for you.

YOU
ARE
ENOUGH

YOU CAN'T LIVE
24 HOURS A DAY
IN THE SPOTLIGHT
AND REMAIN
CREATIVE. FOR
PEOPLE LIKE ME,
SOLITUDE IS
A VICTORY.

KARL LAGERFELD

MAKE IT A MASSAGE

Tense muscles can cause stress and drain your energy. So, if you've got the budget, book yourself in for a massage. Even just a short Indian head massage can work wonders for your mood and leave you feeling rejuvenated. If you can't make it to a treatment room, try a self-massage. Recreate a peaceful environment with no harsh lights or loud sounds, then light candles and add essential oils with calming fragrances. There are plenty of techniques for self-massage explained online and just a few minutes of looking after yourself will make a difference to how you're feeling.

COMPARISON IS THE THIEF OF JOY

If only there were a magic wand that we could wave to stop us comparing ourselves to other people, whether on social media, at work or in our personal lives. It's one thing to know that comparison really is a waste of time, but another to figure out how to stop doing it. Being aware of who you compare yourself to is a great place to start. Remember, most people will only reveal a small part of their life. Often, underneath it all, they are simply feeling their way through life just like you are. Acknowledge you might not know the full story behind a social media post and that comparing yourself to others is really quite futile and will only make you feel more isolated. Each time you find yourself likening yourself to someone else, flip it around to compare yourself to *you*. How far have you come in the past five years? What have you learned and achieved? How have you grown, both emotionally and socially? As your sense of self-worth grows, you'll find your need for comparison will dwindle.

Love your own company

People who are happy in their own company experience increased feelings of happiness and satisfaction and are better at stress management, so why not learn to be your own best friend? View spending time alone as a good thing – when you can look after your own needs without having to compromise. Start the process by taking yourself out to enjoy some of your favourite things, whether that's seeing a film, enjoying a meal out or planning an activity. Value that precious time alone and continue to schedule in time for yourself once a week.

LONELINESS ADDS
BEAUTY TO LIFE.
IT PUTS A SPECIAL
BURN ON SUNSETS
AND MAKES NIGHT
AIR SMELL BETTER.

HENRY ROLLINS

Sometimes you have to stand alone just to make sure you still can

Do what you want

It's time to focus on you and doing what makes you happy. It sounds simple, but it can take a lot of practice. When you really look at what it is you want to do with your free time and follow your interests, you'll soon find yourself with like-minded people and friendships will start to grow organically. So, start living the life you want today.

PHONE A FRIEND

While you might not always be able to physically see your best friend, be sure to pick up your phone and make a call when you're feeling lonely. Even if your chat lasts just a few minutes or you only get through to their answerphone – make sure you leave a message – you'll feel that boost from a real-life connection.

Loneliness isn't a final destination

IT'S EASY TO STAND
IN THE CROWD BUT IT
TAKES COURAGE TO
STAND ALONE.

MAHATMA GANDHI

ATTRACT THE GOOD STUFF

An affirmation is a positive statement that you repeat in order to combat negative thoughts and feelings. It might feel a bit silly at first, but this repetitiveness can really lift your mood, help boost your self-esteem and ease stress and depression. First, find the positive affirmation that you need to hear. Then, look in the mirror and repeat the sentence confidently to yourself five times. If you're struggling to find the right affirmation, you're in luck as this book is crammed with positive statements that you can repeat as often as you need. You can do this!

SORT OUT YOUR SOCIALS

Keeping your social platforms friendly and kind will work wonders for a positive outlook. Even better, they can be used to interact with people who help you feel comfortable and happy in yourself. Here are a few tips to help you manage your online media.

DO have a regular edit of people you follow or who follow you.

DON'T follow anyone who makes you feel bad about yourself.

DO monitor how much time you are spending online.

DON'T believe everything you see on social media – people use filters and don't always tell the truth.

DO feel free to interact with communities that share your interests.

DON'T believe fake news – check if facts and stats are true using a trusted news source.

DO think about what you're posting – only share information you feel comfortable with.

DON'T make unkind comments online – you don't know what a person is going through.

DO have a social media break every few weeks just for a day or two.

Find your funny side

Laugh and the world laughs with you... because laughter is contagious. And even if you start by fake laughing, chances are that you'll end up in genuine fits of giggles before too long. Laughing, as long as you're not being unkind, is a great way to bond with people you don't know very well and create more meaningful connections. In fact, experts suggest "laughter yoga" – a process where you combine deep breathing exercises with laughing heartily – as a way of keeping healthy while having fun. So next time the opportunity comes along, don't hold back – show your funny side.

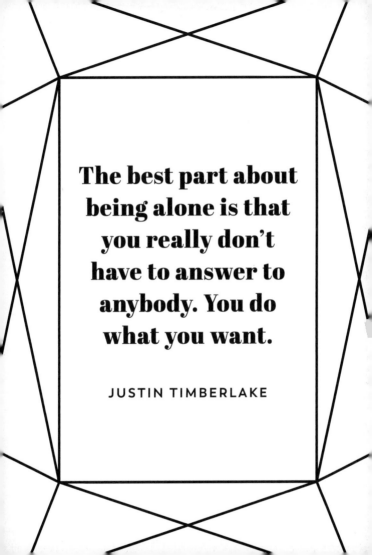

The best part about being alone is that you really don't have to answer to anybody. You do what you want.

JUSTIN TIMBERLAKE

LAUGHTER LEADS
TO GOOD TIMES
AND BEAUTIFUL
MEMORIES

BE KIND...

... to yourself. It's all too easy to put yourself down or give yourself a hard time when things don't go to plan but see if you can get in the habit of treating yourself with compassion instead. Imagine the positive words you would say to a friend in similar circumstances and offer yourself the same upbeat self-talk. Give yourself plenty of time, love and self-compassion because the more you do it, the easier it becomes – making self-kindness a habit you'll want to keep.

Escape with a film

If you're feeling a bit lost and lonely, allow yourself to switch off for a couple of hours. Try snuggling on the sofa and putting on your favourite film. While it's not a permanent fix, it can help you escape from a rabbit hole of negativity for an hour or two. When the end credits roll, you should feel more relaxed and positive and ready to re-enter real life again.

I MAY BE ALONE,
BUT I DON'T HAVE
TO BE LONELY

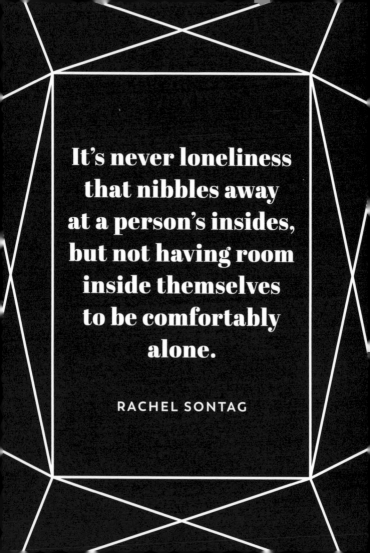

It's never loneliness that nibbles away at a person's insides, but not having room inside themselves to be comfortably alone.

RACHEL SONTAG

WRITE YOUR OWN STORY

When you have lots of thoughts going through your head, it can be soothing to empty them out onto a blank page. Keeping a daily journal, or an occasional one, encourages positivity and helps to avoid negative thoughts. As well as writing down your feelings, try adding three things you're grateful for that day. This healthy outlook will eventually seep off the page and into your real life, helping you to move forward, invigorated and with purpose.

Hold on to the truth

Sometimes, feelings of loneliness can lead you to believe your own narrative – especially any negative thoughts you may be experiencing. When this happens, it's even more important to challenge that negativity you have about yourself and others. Start by questioning if a so-called "fact" is true. Did the new person at work really snub you or could it be that they didn't hear your greeting? Is your friend ignoring your messages or are they just really busy and haven't found time to text you back? Was an invitation not extended to you intentionally, or could that person simply not have realized you might be interested and available? Look for the evidence for your negative beliefs – and if there is none, err on the side of compassion. Not harbouring such negative thoughts will allow you to be open to positive interactions. Remember, most people are rarely unpleasant on purpose. Think the best of people and you might be agreeably surprised.

PICTURE
YOUR DREAMS

One of the best things about having plenty of time by yourself is that you have time to put your ambitions into motion. Try creating a mood board to reflect your hopes and dreams for the future. Maybe you're planning a big renovation for your home, or you have a dream list of travel destinations. Whatever it is, cut out pictures, doodle or paint colours that reflect these goals. Collate them in a scrapbook or on a big piece of paper. Then whenever you're feeling a bit low, refer back to your board for guidance and inspiration.

BUILDING CONNECTIONS

It might seem like a simple solution, but when you're feeling lonely, trying to build connections can be harder than you might think. But that's okay. There's no need to give up or lose confidence. You just need to find the people who you get on with and who also *get* you. This chapter is crammed full of ideas to help you create new social networks and strengthen the ones you already have.

BOOST YOUR SOCIAL SKILLS

The following tips can help you improve your ability to hold a conversation, allowing you to fully immerse in the interactions you encounter:

1   Learn to actively listen. This means not simply waiting for your turn to speak but making sure you really understand what the other person is saying. Silence is golden. Give the person who is speaking your undivided attention and try to be non-judgemental.

2   Look for non-verbal cues such as eye contact, nodding, smiling and mirroring. This shows the person you're talking to is immersed in your interaction. Likewise, you can return these cues to show you're engaged in the conversation.

3   Sustain eye contact. Nerves can make you look around when you're conversing with someone, but it can be really off-putting to the person you're with.

4   Speak slowly. It can be tempting to rush your words when you're feeling nervous, but this can create an even more awkward situation if you're asked to repeat yourself.

5   Pause at the end of each sentence to deliberately slow down your speech. It might sound strange to your ear, but the other person will barely notice.

Fill your diary

Like attracts like, so think about what you're interested in. For example, many people find music to be uplifting, so if you enjoy live music, why not see whether any good bands are playing near you? Spending the evening dancing to great tunes will make you feel connected even if you don't speak to anyone. Or perhaps there is a new art gallery or theatre show in town. Being among fellow music enthusiasts or art fans will provide you with a common talking point. Keep an eye on local Facebook groups or bulletin boards for anything new and interesting.

Better to be alone than surrounded by toxicity

GET EDUCATED

If you've always fancied learning a new language or wanted to try your hand at a skill, such as pottery for example, now is the time to find a course near you. There are a whole host of evening classes available either online or in person – and most are great places to make connections with those who share the same goals as you. Bear in mind that other students are often also looking for more than just an education – and you are likely to meet people who are willing to go out for a quick drink or something to eat when the class is over.

IT'S BETTER TO
HAVE NOBODY,
THAN TO HAVE
SOMEONE WHO
IS HALF THERE,
OR DOESN'T
WANT TO
BE THERE.

ANGELINA JOLIE

Believe in yourself and you will be unstoppable

JOIN A
BOOK CLUB

Who doesn't love chatting about their
favourite book? If you're keen to make
connections, join a local book club. It can either
be virtual or in person, and it's the perfect
reason to come together with a group of like-
minded people. If there aren't any book clubs
in your area, you could set one up yourself. Put
a poster up in your local library or advertise
it on social media. You'll hopefully soon hear
from fellow bookworms. The only hard part
will be choosing which book to discuss.

DON'T WAIT
FOR OTHERS TO
GIVE YOU WHAT
YOU WANT,
GO AND GET IT
FOR YOURSELF

Be a team player

One effective way to tackle feelings of loneliness is to join a local sports team. It doesn't matter which sport you choose or if you're any good at it – the people at the club will all have different abilities, so don't let your lack of skills stop you from taking part. Whether it's a local running group, soccer club or netball team that piques your interest, all you need to do is sign up. After a few sessions, when you're feeling more comfortable with your teammates, you'll feel confident enough to attend post-training drinks and other social events.

YOU NEED TO KNOW HOW TO BE ALONE AND NOT BE DEFINED BY ANOTHER PERSON.

OSCAR WILDE

MAKE
SPACE FOR
LONELINESS

HELP OTHERS

Some days it might feel as though you don't have enough fuel in the tank to look after yourself, let alone help somebody else – but giving back to the community is one of the most positive things you can do to give yourself a boost. Volunteering increases your self-esteem, eases depression and lowers anxiety. So, whether you sign up with an organization or charity or commit to helping a neighbour with their shopping once a week, doing things for someone else can really help to enhance your sense of belonging and well-being. Not only will you feel more positive, but you'll also feel part of a community of helpers, and you never know what friendships might form as you meet new people. If you're not sure where to start, a simple internet search should put you in touch with some organizations in your area. Or pop into your local library, town hall or religious building to find out about volunteering opportunities.

Find online friends

If you're struggling to make connections in real life, turn to the power of the internet. Aside from social media groups, there are "find a friend" websites that work like dating websites, but you're matched with potential friends instead of partners. However, you still need to keep a cool head and remember not to put yourself in any danger when meeting up with potential new buddies. Always tell someone where you're going and with whom. And don't neglect real-life friendship opportunities just because you're trying to meet people online. Stay open to all opportunities!

PEOPLE ARE NEVER
TOO OLD OR TOO
YOUNG TO LOOK
FOR HUMAN
CONNECTION.

JOHN TURTURRO

Looking for love

Sometimes the connections we're longing for are more than just friendships. If you're looking for love, there are plenty of places where you can meet a partner. Hobby clubs and classes are great places to meet people who enjoy the same activities as you, and dating apps and websites are readily available. If you choose the latter, remember to be cautious about who you agree to meet. People can often pretend to be someone else online, so always tell a friend where you're going and who you're meeting.

Starting off with a daytime date, such as a coffee meeting or lunch, before moving on to a dinner date is another way of slowly getting to know a potential love interest. Allow your relationship to progress at a pace you feel comfortable with. Red flags to look out for include someone who is not forthcoming with information about their life or who asks if they can borrow money. If you are ever in doubt, follow your instincts and cancel.

I THINK IT'S GOOD FOR
A PERSON TO SPEND
TIME ALONE. IT GIVES
THEM AN OPPORTUNITY
TO DISCOVER
WHO THEY ARE.

AMY SEDARIS

MAKE
TIME FOR
YOURSELF
TODAY

WALK AND TALK

Registering with a walking club is a great way to get out of your comfort zone and meet new people. At the very least, you'll discover more about your local area – and even if you've been living somewhere for years, it's guaranteed to open your eyes to something new. At most, you could form meaningful bonds that could last a lifetime. In fact, counsellors often suggest "walking and talking therapy" as a beautiful way to connect with people while doing something pleasant and enjoyable. After all, it's nearly impossible not to fall into step and start chatting with someone when you're on a hike. Plus, you'll be keeping fit and healthy while you mingle. Just make sure to invest in comfortable weatherproof clothing and shoes as it's hard to make friends when you're soaking wet or worrying about blisters. Look online for walking groups near you or ask in a local outdoor activities store for advice on nearby trails.

REIGNITE OLD FRIENDSHIPS

While it's great to make new friends, consider getting in touch with chums who you haven't seen for a while. Think about those who you loved hanging out with but who gradually faded from your life for various reasons, such as work commitments or moving away. You don't need to overthink it: dropping someone a friendly message to see how they are and saying you'd love to meet up is the perfect way to reconnect. Continue to steer clear of any toxic friends. The chances are they haven't changed their ways and you're better off without them.

YOU DO NOT
NEED THE
COMPANY OF
OTHERS TO FEEL
HAPPINESS

SOLO HOLIDAYS

It can feel quite daunting to head off on vacation alone, so if you're not quite ready for a solo adventure, consider talking to a travel operator who specializes in singles' holidays. Ask for an itinerary that encompasses your interests, such as taking in culture, nature experiences or outdoor escapades. Do your research to find a reputable organizer and get ready for the adventure of a lifetime. By choosing a bespoke holiday, you will probably meet like-minded travellers. You might even find someone you'd like to travel with regularly.

NOWHERE IS
IT WRITTEN
THAT YOU
CAN'T DO IT.

ELENA FERRANTE

Being surrounded by the wrong people is the loneliest thing in the world

Get involved

All around you, community projects are crying out for your help. Consider stopping off at your local library and offering to help out on your free evenings. Try speaking to a few community groups, via your local church or aged-care centre, about serving tea and cake at their next get-together. Creating that bond or camaraderie with a nearby network can not only make a difference to the community, but also you'll get to meet more people in your local area.

YOU'RE ALWAYS
WITH YOURSELF SO YOU
MIGHT AS WELL ENJOY
THE COMPANY.

DIANE VON
FURSTENBERG

No matter how dark it gets, the sun is still going to rise

BORROW A DOG

It's widely considered that a four-legged friend is the ideal partner but owning a dog is a big commitment – so why not borrow one instead? Ask friends or family if they could do with a dog-sitter, or a brief online search will lead you to owners looking for people to dog-sit during the day while they're at work or on weekends if they're away. No one can resist stroking a dog when they see one out and about, so you'll meet lots of new people and get VIP access to your local dog-walking community – all you have to do is show up at your local park with a happy hound. Best of all, stroking a dog on a regular basis helps to reduce anxiety as well as enhance thinking skills – so hanging out with a dog can help to reduce any fear you have around social situations, too.

THE MORE
HAPPINESS
YOU GIVE,
THE MORE YOU
GET IN RETURN

KEEP SIGHT OF YOURSELF

When you're busy trying to build connections, you're bound to experience some rejections. Stay grounded by reminding yourself that the person in question may be dealing with something that you know nothing about, which may be why they couldn't connect with you at that time. If you find your confidence wavering, write yourself a love list of all your great qualities. If you're struggling to come up with options, ask a loved one to help you out. Their answers may surprise you, but you'll get the boost you need to get back out there and make friends.

Just say yes

It can be easy to fall into a habit of saying "no" to new events and activities, especially when nerves get in the way. This inhibition, however, can mean that you're not connecting with people to your full potential, which in turn can lead to those feelings of loneliness.

Consider making a conscious decision to say "yes" to the majority of opportunities that come along. Okay, you might feel a little overwhelmed at first but taking it a step at a time will help. Start with saying "yes" to something out of your comfort zone once a month. Then, expand this to twice a month, then once a week and so on. Remember, the choice to go out is still in your hands – and this is a powerful step forward in helping reduce the negativity you have been feeling. Take your time and see how a positive "why not?" attitude can lead you to meeting interesting people.

ROLE PLAY

It can be intimidating to start up a conversation with someone new, but that doesn't mean you shouldn't try. Practise in advance by asking a trusted friend or family member if they'll help you with some role play. They could pose as a stranger in a night class or café to see if you can strike up a conversation with them. Perhaps they can even meet you in a coffee shop and pretend not to know you. Try different scenarios in different places and have some fun with it –

changing the conversation depending on what you wish to talk about that day. It might feel strange at first, but you'll soon find yourself improving those opening gambits, and you'll have a few stock sentences that will come in handy when you're facing a real-life situation. Remember, these things rarely come naturally to anyone, but the more you do it, the better you'll get and the less scary it will feel. So, go for it!

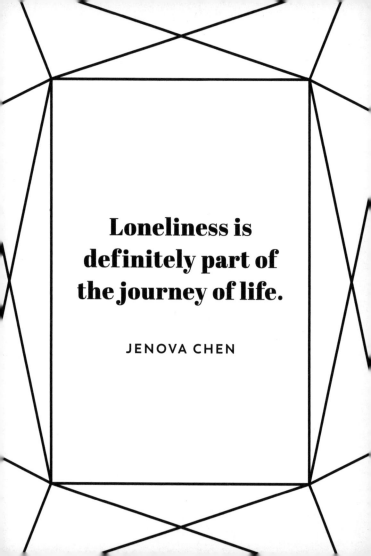

Loneliness is definitely part of the journey of life.

JENOVA CHEN

DO NOT GIVE
YOUR PAST THE
POWER TO DEFINE
YOUR FUTURE

GETTING PROFESSIONAL HELP

Sometimes the weight of loneliness becomes so heavy, you can't carry it alone. If this is the case, it is important to reach out for professional help. Of course, friends and family can be incredibly supportive if you find yourself struggling, but sometimes expert assistance will make a bigger difference. Remember, visiting your doctor, a trained counsellor or psychotherapist isn't a sign of weakness, it's a phenomenal sign of strength that you refuse to give up.

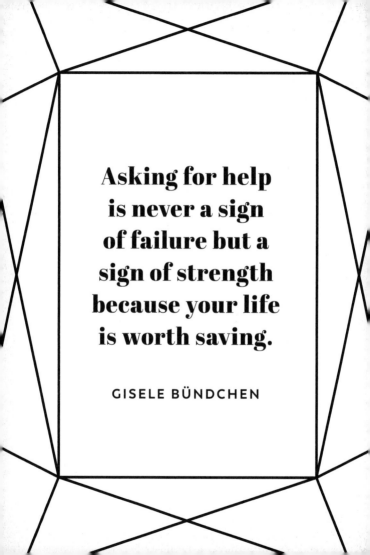

TAKING THE
FIRST STEP

It can feel overwhelming to reach out for help, especially if you're used to bottling up your emotions. So, start small. Why not write a diary or a journal that talks openly about how you're feeling? This can double up as a prompt when you seek help from a doctor or therapist. If the thought of confiding in a stranger feels too much, ask a trusted friend or family member if you could practise talking about your feelings with them first. It might feel as if your words will stay lodged in your throat, but the more you talk about your worries and problems, the easier it gets.

Your feelings of loneliness matter, and you'd be surprised at how many people feel the same way. Often loneliness goes hand in hand with other issues such as low self-esteem, anxiety and depression. This is nothing to be ashamed of, and the more you speak about it, the sooner you'll be able to work on the issues you're struggling with.

IF YOU ARE NEVER
ALONE, YOU
CANNOT KNOW
YOURSELF.

PAULO COELHO

Professionally speaking

Your doctor will be able to provide you with the details of local charities and support groups that you might find useful. If you're not ready to talk further, you can call or email a helpline from the comfort and security of your home. Charities such as the Samaritans offer 24-hour helplines that you can call day or night, if you feel overwhelmed or distressed. Bear in mind that some people find talking to a stranger easier than confiding in a friend or family member. Although you might feel alone right now, rest assured there are people out there waiting to help you.

Reframe
your thoughts

Cognitive Behaviour Therapy (CBT) is designed to change the way you think and behave when confronted with problems, and it can also help when trying to negotiate your way through the negative thoughts that often come with loneliness. Typically practised with a trained counsellor, CBT will help you break down your worries into smaller, more manageable chunks, change your negative thought patterns into constructive considerations and find practical ways to improve your state of mind.

While it's best to work with an experienced CBT professional, you can adopt some of the practices yourself. Start by examining your negative thoughts. Do you dwell on the minor details or always assume the worst? Once you're aware of your tendencies, you will be in a position to recognize this behaviour when it happens and consciously reframe your negative thinking. Start small and be kind to yourself. There are plenty of books or podcasts that can help you learn CBT techniques if you aren't ready for professional therapy right now.

THERE IS NOTHING
OUTSIDE OF
YOURSELF,
LOOK WITHIN.
EVERYTHING YOU
WANT IS THERE.

RUMI

It won't always feel this hard

DON'T GIVE UP

When we feel utterly alone, it can seem as if there is no point going on. But even in those moments when it feels as though you're wading through emotional distress, it's important to remember these feelings do pass. However bad you feel now, it hasn't always been this difficult, and if you can stay strong, you will find better times again. Bear in mind that without the dark, it's harder to appreciate the light. And despite how it may seem, no one is happy all the time.

If you're feeling really low, avoid making any drastic decisions. Call a family member or trusted friend and ask them to come and be with you. Even if you sit in silence, simply knowing you have someone close can relieve a lot of the strain. If you need to, call the emergency services and explain you need immediate help. Think of your feelings like waves. They will rise and crash, but you don't have to surf them all.

It's okay to try again tomorrow

YOU HAVE TO GO
AHEAD, EVEN IF NO
ONE GOES WITH YOU.

LAILAH GIFTY AKITA

CONCLUSION

The very fact this book exists means that there are plenty of people dealing with feelings of loneliness. So, while you may feel alone, you really aren't. In order to change your life, you must be brave and make some changes to your attitude and your actions. For example, see if you can reframe your feelings and thoughts and think about all the friends you haven't met yet. Take those chances, say "yes" to opportunities and let the world see who you are. By deciding to take this step forward, you're choosing to change your life. Hopefully, the advice in this book can guide you on your path to happiness. All you need to do is keep moving forward, and you'll get there in the end.

RESOURCES

For readers in the United Kingdom:

Volunteering:
Visit www.reachvolunteering.org.uk for nationwide volunteering opportunities

Anxiety UK: This charity provides information, support and understanding for those living with anxiety disorders. www.anxietyuk.org.uk

Mind: A mental health charity offering support and advice to help empower anyone experiencing mental health concerns. www.mind.org.uk

Samaritans: A 24-hour, free, confidential helpline, to support you whatever you're going through. www.samaritans.org; call 116 123; or email jo@samaritans.org (UK) or jo@samaritans.ie (Ireland)

SANEline: A national, out-of-hours mental health helpline: www.sane.org.uk; call 0300 304 7000 (4.30p.m.–10.30p.m.); or email support@sane.org.uk

For readers in the United States:

Find volunteer opportunities: www.oneworld365.org

Freedom From Fear: A national non-profit mental health advocacy organization, helping to positively impact the lives of all those affected by anxiety, depression and related disorders. www.freedomfromfear.org

Mental Health America: promoting the overall mental health of all Americans. www.mhanational.org

Mental Health Foundation: A non-profit organization specializing in mental health awareness, education, suicide prevention and addiction. mentalhealthfoundation.org

National Suicide Prevention Line: A 24/7 free, confidential support service for those in distress, as well as crisis resources for loved ones. www.suicidepreventionlifeline.org; or call 1-800-273-8255

If you're interested in finding out more about our books, find us on Facebook at **Summersdale Publishers**, on Twitter at **@Summersdale** and on Instagram at **@summersdalebooks** and get in touch. We'd love to hear from you!

Thank you very much for buying this Summersdale book.

www.summersdale.com